Lupus Recovery
Diet Cookbook

Anti-Inflammatory Recipes for Reduced Inflammation, Improved Immune Function, and Better Health."

Judy Kelly

Table of Contents

Introduction

Welcome to the "Lupus Recovery Diet Cookbook," a labor of love crafted to support you on your journey to health and wellness. Living with lupus presents its challenges, but by embracing the healing power of food, we can nourish our bodies and nurture our spirits.

I understand the complexities of living with lupus, from the uncertainty of flare-ups to the fatigue that can be all-consuming. That's why I've created this cookbook—to offer you a collection of recipes that not only taste delicious but also support your well-being.

This cookbook is more than just a collection of recipes; it's a celebration of resilience and strength. It's a reminder that you are not alone on this journey. Together, we can embrace the healing power of food and nourish our bodies from the inside out.

As you explore the recipes in this cookbook, I encourage you to listen to your body and honor its needs. Each recipe is crafted with care, using ingredients that are not only delicious but also thoughtfully selected to support your health.

I hope this cookbook inspires you to get creative in the kitchen and discover new ways to enjoy the foods that support your well-being. May these recipes bring you joy, comfort, and nourishment as you continue on your path to healing.

Thank you for allowing me to be a part of your journey. Here's to good health, delicious food, and the healing power of the Lupus Recovery Diet.

With love and gratitude,
Judy

Understanding Lupus and the Benefits of the Lupus Recovery Diet

What is Lupus?

Lupus is a chronic autoimmune disease that can affect various parts of the body, including the skin, joints, kidneys, heart, and brain. In lupus, the immune system becomes overactive and attacks healthy tissues, leading to inflammation, pain, and damage to organs.

How Does Diet Affect Lupus?

Diet plays a crucial role in managing lupus symptoms and improving overall health. Certain foods can trigger inflammation and worsen symptoms, while others can help reduce inflammation and promote healing.

Benefits of the Lupus Recovery Diet

1. Reduced Inflammation: The Lupus Recovery Diet focuses on anti-inflammatory foods, such as fruits, vegetables, whole grains, and healthy fats. These foods can help reduce inflammation in the body, which is beneficial for managing lupus symptoms.

2. Improved Immune Function: The diet includes foods that support a healthy immune system, such as those rich in vitamins, minerals, and antioxidants. A strong immune system is important for managing lupus and reducing the risk of infections.

3. Better Digestive Health: Many of the foods included in the Lupus Recovery Diet are beneficial for gut health, such as fiber-rich fruits and vegetables and probiotic-rich foods like yogurt. A healthy gut can improve digestion and nutrient absorption.

4. Weight Management: The diet emphasizes whole, nutrient-dense foods and limits processed foods and sugars, which can help individuals maintain a healthy weight. This is important for managing lupus and reducing the risk of obesity-related complications.

5. Increased Energy Levels: By providing the body with the nutrients it needs, the Lupus Recovery Diet can help improve energy levels, reducing fatigue, which is a common symptom of lupus.

6. Improved Mood and Mental Health: Some foods included in the diet, such as fatty fish rich in omega-3 fatty acids, are known to have mood-boosting properties. A healthy diet can also improve mental clarity and overall well-being.

How This Cookbook Can Help You

This cookbook is a valuable resource for anyone looking to manage their lupus symptoms and improve their overall health through diet. Here's how this cookbook can help you:

1. Nutrient-Rich Recipes: The cookbook offers a wide range of nutrient-rich recipes specifically designed to support the lupus recovery process. These recipes are packed with vitamins, minerals, and antioxidants to help reduce inflammation and promote healing.

2. Easy-to-Follow Meal Plans: The cookbook includes easy-to-follow meal plans that take the guesswork out of meal planning. Whether you're looking for a quick and easy breakfast or a satisfying dinner, the meal plans provide delicious and nutritious options for every meal.

3. Variety of Recipes: From comforting soups to hearty main dishes and delicious desserts, this cookbook offers a variety of recipes to suit every taste and craving. Each recipe is carefully crafted to be both delicious and nutritious, making it easy to stick to your lupus recovery diet.

4. Education and Information: In addition to recipes, the cookbook also provides education and information about the lupus recovery diet. You'll learn about the principles of the diet, foods to include and avoid, and tips for success on the diet.

5. Empowerment: By following the recipes in this cookbook, you'll be taking control of your health and empowering yourself to live your best life with lupus. The recipes are designed to nourish your body and support your overall well-being, helping you feel your best every day.

Overall, this cookbook is a comprehensive guide to the lupus recovery diet, offering delicious recipes, helpful meal plans, and valuable information to support you on your journey to health and wellness.

Chapter 1: The Basics of the Lupus Recovery Diet

What is the Lupus Recovery Diet?

The Lupus Recovery Diet is a dietary approach specifically designed to help individuals with lupus manage their symptoms and improve their overall health. It focuses on consuming foods that are known to reduce inflammation, support the immune system, and promote overall well-being.

Key principles of the Lupus Recovery Diet include:

1. Anti-Inflammatory Foods: The diet emphasizes foods that are rich in antioxidants and anti-inflammatory compounds, such as fruits, vegetables, whole grains, nuts, seeds, and fatty fish.

2. Healthy Fats: Healthy fats, such as those found in olive oil, avocados, and nuts, are an important part of the diet. These fats help reduce inflammation and support brain health.

3. Lean Proteins: Lean protein sources, such as chicken, turkey, and legumes, are included in moderation to support muscle health and immune function.

4. Limiting Processed Foods: Processed foods, sugary snacks, and beverages are limited or avoided, as they can contribute to inflammation and worsen lupus symptoms.

5. Hydration: Staying hydrated is important for overall health, so the diet encourages drinking plenty of water and avoiding sugary drinks.

6. Individualized Approach: The Lupus Recovery Diet is not a one-size-fits-all approach. It can be tailored to meet individual needs and preferences, taking into account any specific dietary restrictions or sensitivities.

Overall, the Lupus Recovery Diet aims to provide individuals with lupus the nutrients they need to support their health and well-being while reducing foods that may trigger inflammation or worsen symptoms.

Principles of the Lupus Recovery Diet

The principles of the Lupus Recovery Diet are based on the idea of using food as a tool to manage lupus symptoms and promote overall health. Here are the key principles of the diet:

1. Anti-Inflammatory Foods: The diet focuses on consuming foods that are known to reduce inflammation in the body. This includes foods rich in antioxidants, such as fruits, vegetables, nuts, seeds, and fatty fish.

2. Balanced Nutrition: The diet aims to provide the body with the nutrients it needs to function optimally. This includes a balance of carbohydrates, protein, and healthy fats, as well as vitamins, minerals, and other essential nutrients.

3. Whole Foods: The diet emphasizes whole, unprocessed foods and avoids or limits processed foods, sugary snacks, and beverages. Whole foods are rich in nutrients and free from additives and preservatives that can contribute to inflammation.

4. Hydration: Staying hydrated is important for overall health and can help flush out toxins from the body. The diet encourages drinking plenty of water and avoiding sugary drinks.

5. Mindful Eating: The diet encourages mindful eating practices, such as paying attention to hunger and fullness cues, eating slowly, and savoring each bite. This can help prevent overeating and promote digestion.

6. Personalized Approach: The Lupus Recovery Diet is not a one-size-fits-all approach. It can be tailored to meet individual needs and

preferences, taking into account any specific dietary restrictions or sensitivities.

By following these principles, individuals with lupus can create a diet that supports their health and well-being, reduces inflammation, and helps manage their symptoms.

Benefits of Following the Lupus Recovery Diet

Following the Lupus Recovery Diet can offer several benefits for individuals with lupus:

1. Reduced Inflammation: The diet focuses on anti-inflammatory foods, which can help reduce inflammation in the body, a key factor in lupus symptom management.

2. Improved Immune Function: By providing the body with essential nutrients, the diet can support a healthier immune system, which is important for individuals with lupus.

3. Better Digestive Health: Many of the foods included in the diet are beneficial for gut health, which can improve digestion and nutrient absorption, supporting overall health.

4. Weight Management: The diet emphasizes whole, nutrient-dense foods and limits processed foods and sugars, which can help individuals maintain a healthy weight, important for managing certain symptoms of lupus.

5. Increased Energy Levels: By providing the body with the nutrients it needs, the diet can help improve energy levels, reducing fatigue, a common symptom of lupus.

6. Improved Mood and Mental Health: Some foods included in the diet are known to have mood-boosting properties, which can help improve mental health and well-being.

Overall, the Lupus Recovery Diet aims to support overall health and well-being for individuals with lupus, helping them manage their symptoms and improve their quality of life.

Chapter 2: Getting Started with the Lupus Recovery Diet

How to Shop for Lupus-Friendly Ingredients

When shopping for lupus-friendly ingredients, it's important to focus on whole, nutrient-dense foods that can help reduce inflammation and support overall health. Here are some tips for shopping for lupus-friendly ingredients:

1. Focus on Fresh Produce: Choose a variety of colorful fruits and vegetables, as they are rich in antioxidants and vitamins that can help reduce inflammation. Aim to include a rainbow of colors in your diet.

2. Choose Lean Proteins: Opt for lean protein sources such as poultry, fish, legumes, and tofu. These foods are rich in protein and can help support muscle health and immune function.

3. Include Healthy Fats: Incorporate sources of healthy fats into your diet, such as olive oil, avocado, nuts, and seeds. These fats can help reduce inflammation and support heart health.

4. Limit Processed Foods: Try to avoid or limit processed foods, sugary snacks, and beverages, as they can contribute to inflammation and worsen lupus symptoms.

5. Read Labels: When shopping for packaged foods, read the labels carefully to avoid ingredients that may trigger inflammation, such as added sugars, trans fats, and artificial additives.

6. Choose Whole Grains: Opt for whole grains such as brown rice, quinoa, oats, and whole wheat bread. These foods are rich in fiber and nutrients that can support digestive health and reduce inflammation.

7. Consider Organic Options: If possible, choose organic fruits and vegetables to reduce exposure to pesticides and other chemicals that may contribute to inflammation.

By focusing on these tips when shopping, you can create a diet that supports your overall health and well-being while managing lupus symptoms.

Tips for Success on the Lupus Recovery Diet

1. Educate Yourself: Learn about the principles of the Lupus Recovery Diet and why certain foods are beneficial or harmful. Understanding the diet can help you make informed choices.

2. Plan Your Meals: Take the time to plan your meals and snacks in advance. This can help you ensure you have the right ingredients on hand and avoid temptation to eat foods that are not part of the diet.

3. Shop Wisely: Use shopping lists and stick to them to avoid purchasing foods that are not part of the Lupus Recovery Diet. Consider shopping at farmers' markets or health food stores for fresh, whole foods.

4. Prepare Your Own Meals: Cooking at home allows you to control the ingredients and ensure that your meals align with the Lupus Recovery Diet. Experiment with new recipes to keep things interesting.

5. Stay Hydrated: Drink plenty of water throughout the day to stay hydrated. Proper hydration is important for overall health and can help reduce inflammation.

6. Listen to Your Body: Pay attention to how your body responds to different foods. Keep a food diary to track your symptoms and identify any foods that may trigger flare-ups.

7. Seek Support: Joining a support group or working with a dietitian who is familiar with the Lupus Recovery Diet can provide you with additional guidance and support.

8. Be Patient: It may take time to see the full benefits of the Lupus Recovery Diet. Be patient with yourself and celebrate small victories along the way.

By following these tips, you can increase your chances of success on the Lupus Recovery Diet and improve your overall health and well-being.

Chapter 3: Anti-Inflammatory Breakfast Recipes

1. OVERNIGHT OATS

Ingredients:
- 1/2 cup rolled oats
- 1/2 cup almond milk
- 1 tablespoon chia seeds
- 1 teaspoon honey
- Fresh berries for topping

Instructions:
1. In a jar, combine oats, almond milk, chia seeds, and honey.
2. Stir well, cover, and refrigerate overnight.
3. In the morning, stir and top with fresh berries before serving.

---

2. GREEK YOGURT PARFAIT

Ingredients:
- 1 cup Greek yogurt
- 1 tablespoon honey
- 1/4 cup granola
- 1/4 cup mixed berries

Instructions:
1. In a bowl or glass, layer Greek yogurt, honey, granola, and mixed berries.
2. Repeat layers.
3. Serve immediately.

—

3. BANANA ALMOND SMOOTHIE

Ingredients:
- 1 ripe banana
- 2 tablespoons almond butter
- 1 cup almond milk
- 1 teaspoon honey
- Ice cubes (optional)

Instructions:
1. In a blender, combine banana, almond butter, almond milk, honey, and ice cubes.
2. Blend until smooth.
3. Pour into a glass and serve immediately.

---

4. SCRAMBLED TOFU

Ingredients:
- 1/2 block firm tofu, crumbled
- 1/4 teaspoon turmeric
- 1/4 teaspoon garlic powder
- 1/4 teaspoon onion powder
- Handful of spinach
- Handful of cherry tomatoes, halved
- Salt and pepper to taste
- Olive oil for cooking

Instructions:
1. In a pan, heat olive oil over medium heat.
2. Add crumbled tofu, turmeric, garlic powder, onion powder, salt, and pepper.
3. Cook for 5-7 minutes, stirring occasionally.
4. Add spinach and cherry tomatoes, and cook until spinach is wilted.

5. Serve hot.

---

5. CHIA SEED PUDDING

Ingredients:
- 2 tablespoons chia seeds
- 1/2 cup coconut milk
- 1/2 teaspoon vanilla extract
- 1 teaspoon honey
- Sliced almonds for topping

Instructions:
1. In a bowl, combine chia seeds, coconut milk, vanilla extract, and honey.
2. Stir well, cover, and refrigerate for at least 2 hours or overnight.
3. Stir again before serving, and top with sliced almonds.

---

6. QUINOA BREAKFAST BOWL

Ingredients:
- 1/2 cup cooked quinoa
- 1/2 cup almond milk
- 1/2 teaspoon cinnamon
- 1 tablespoon honey or maple syrup
- Fresh berries and nuts for topping

Instructions:
1. In a small saucepan, heat almond milk over medium heat until warm.
2. Stir in cooked quinoa, cinnamon, and honey or maple syrup.
3. Cook for 2-3 minutes, stirring occasionally, until heated through.
4. Remove from heat and let it sit for a minute.
5. Transfer to a bowl, top with fresh berries and nuts, and serve warm.

7. AVOCADO TOAST WITH POACHED EGG

Ingredients:
- 2 slices whole grain bread, toasted
- 1 ripe avocado, mashed
- 2 eggs
- Salt and pepper to taste
- Red pepper flakes for garnish (optional)

Instructions:
1. Poach the eggs: Bring a pot of water to a simmer, add a splash of vinegar, and gently crack the eggs into the water. Cook for 3-4 minutes until the whites are set but the yolks are still runny. Remove with a slotted spoon and drain on a paper towel.
2. Spread mashed avocado evenly on each slice of toast.
3. Top each with a poached egg.
4. Season with salt, pepper, and red pepper flakes.
5. Serve immediately.

---

8. BERRY SMOOTHIE BOWL

Ingredients:
- 1 cup frozen mixed berries
- 1 banana
- 1/2 cup almond milk
- 1 tablespoon honey or maple syrup
- Granola, nuts, and seeds for topping

Instructions:
1. In a blender, combine frozen berries, banana, almond milk, and honey or maple syrup.
2. Blend until smooth, adding more almond milk if needed.
3. Pour into a bowl and top with granola, nuts, and seeds.

9. APPLE CINNAMON OATMEAL

Ingredients:
- 1/2 cup rolled oats
- 1 cup almond milk
- 1 apple, diced
- 1/2 teaspoon cinnamon
- 1 tablespoon honey or maple syrup

Instructions:
1. In a saucepan, combine oats, almond milk, apple, cinnamon, and honey or maple syrup.
2. Bring to a boil, then reduce heat and simmer for 5-7 minutes, stirring occasionally, until oats are cooked and mixture is thickened.
3. Remove from heat and let it sit for a minute.
4. Serve hot.

---

10. SPINACH AND MUSHROOM OMELETTE

Ingredients:
- 2 eggs
- 1/4 cup almond milk
- Handful of spinach, chopped
- Handful of mushrooms, sliced
- 1/4 cup grated cheese (optional)
- Salt and pepper to taste
- Olive oil for cooking

Instructions:
1. In a bowl, whisk together eggs, almond milk, salt, and pepper.
2. Heat olive oil in a skillet over medium heat.
3. Add spinach and mushrooms, and cook until spinach is wilted and mushrooms are softened.

4. Pour in the egg mixture, and let it cook for a few minutes until the edges start to set.
5. Sprinkle grated cheese on top, if using, and fold the omelette in half.
6. Cook for another minute or until the cheese is melted and the eggs are cooked through.
7. Serve hot.

---

11. BLUEBERRY BANANA PANCAKES

Ingredients:
- 1/2 cup whole wheat flour
- 1/2 teaspoon baking powder
- 1/4 teaspoon baking soda
- Pinch of salt
- 1/2 cup almond milk
- 1 tablespoon honey or maple syrup
- 1 ripe banana, mashed
- 1/2 cup blueberries

Instructions:
1. In a bowl, whisk together flour, baking powder, baking soda, and salt.
2. In another bowl, mix almond milk, honey or maple syrup, and mashed banana.
3. Pour the wet ingredients into the dry ingredients and stir until just combined.
4. Gently fold in the blueberries.
5. Heat a non-stick skillet over medium heat and lightly grease with oil.
6. Pour 1/4 cup of batter onto the skillet for each pancake.
7. Cook for 2-3 minutes, or until bubbles form on the surface.
8. Flip and cook for another 1-2 minutes, or until golden brown.
9. Serve warm with maple syrup and extra blueberries.

—

12. MANGO COCONUT CHIA PUDDING

Ingredients:
- 2 tablespoons chia seeds
- 1/2 cup coconut milk
- 1/2 teaspoon vanilla extract
- 1 teaspoon honey or maple syrup
- 1/2 cup diced mango
- Shredded coconut for topping

Instructions:
1. In a bowl, combine chia seeds, coconut milk, vanilla extract, and honey or maple syrup.
2. Stir well, cover, and refrigerate for at least 2 hours or overnight.
3. Before serving, top with diced mango and shredded coconut.

---

13. SWEET POTATO BREAKFAST BOWL

Ingredients:
- 1 small sweet potato, roasted and mashed
- 1/2 cup Greek yogurt
- 1 tablespoon almond butter
- 1 tablespoon honey
- Granola for topping

Instructions:
1. In a bowl, layer roasted and mashed sweet potato, Greek yogurt, almond butter, and honey.
2. Top with granola before serving.

—

14. GREEN SMOOTHIE

Ingredients:
- 1 cup spinach
- 1/2 cucumber, chopped
- 1/2 banana
- 1/2 cup almond milk
- 1/2 tablespoon honey or maple syrup

Instructions:
1. In a blender, combine spinach, cucumber, banana, almond milk, and honey or maple syrup.
2. Blend until smooth.
3. Serve immediately.

---

15. BREAKFAST BURRITO

Ingredients:
- 2 eggs, scrambled
- 1/4 cup black beans, drained and rinsed
- 2 tablespoons salsa
- 1 whole wheat tortilla
- 1/4 avocado, sliced

Instructions:
1. In a skillet, scramble the eggs.
2. Warm the tortilla in the skillet.
3. Layer the eggs, black beans, salsa, and avocado slices on the tortilla.
4. Roll up the tortilla to form a burrito.

---

16. PEANUT BUTTER BANANA TOAST

Ingredients:
- 2 slices whole grain bread, toasted
- 2 tablespoons peanut butter
- 1 banana, sliced
- Honey or maple syrup for drizzling

Instructions:
1. Spread peanut butter on each slice of toast.
2. Top with banana slices.
3. Drizzle with honey or maple syrup.

---

17. YOGURT AND FRUIT BOWL

Ingredients:
- 1 cup Greek yogurt
- 1/2 cup mixed berries
- 1 tablespoon honey
- 1/4 cup granola

Instructions:
1. In a bowl, layer Greek yogurt, mixed berries, honey, and granola.
2. Serve chilled.

---

18. BREAKFAST QUINOA

Ingredients:
- 1/2 cup cooked quinoa
- 1/2 cup almond milk
- 1 tablespoon honey

- 1/4 teaspoon cinnamon
- Sliced almonds for topping

Instructions:
1. In a saucepan, combine quinoa, almond milk, honey, and cinnamon.
2. Cook over medium heat until heated through.
3. Top with sliced almonds before serving.

---

19. BREAKFAST SMOOTHIE JAR

Ingredients:
- 1/2 cup oats
- 1/2 cup almond milk
- 1/2 banana
- 1/2 cup mixed berries
- 1 tablespoon chia seeds
- 1 tablespoon almond butter

Instructions:
1. In a jar, layer oats, almond milk, banana, mixed berries, chia seeds, and almond butter.
2. Refrigerate overnight.
3. Stir before eating.

---

20. TOMATO AVOCADO TOAST

Ingredients:
- 2 slices whole grain bread, toasted
- 1/2 avocado, mashed
- 1/2 cup cherry tomatoes, halved
- Salt, pepper, and red pepper flakes to taste

- Olive oil for drizzling

Instructions:
1. Spread mashed avocado on each slice of toast.
2. Top with cherry tomatoes.
3. Season with salt, pepper, and red pepper flakes.
4. Drizzle with olive oil.

Chapter 4: Anti-Inflammatory Lunch Recipes

1. TURMERIC CHICKEN SALAD

Ingredients:
- 1 chicken breast, cooked and shredded
- 1/2 teaspoon turmeric
- 1/4 teaspoon garlic powder
- 1/4 teaspoon onion powder
- Salt and pepper to taste
- 2 cups mixed greens
- 1/2 cucumber, sliced
- 1/2 bell pepper, sliced
- 1/4 cup cherry tomatoes, halved
- 2 tablespoons olive oil
- 1 tablespoon apple cider vinegar
- 1/2 tablespoon honey

Instructions:
1. In a bowl, combine shredded chicken with turmeric, garlic powder, onion powder, salt, and pepper.
2. In another bowl, mix olive oil, apple cider vinegar, and honey to make the dressing.
3. In a large bowl, combine mixed greens, cucumber, bell pepper, and cherry tomatoes.
4. Top with seasoned chicken and drizzle with dressing.

---

2. QUINOA STUFFED BELL PEPPERS

Ingredients:
- 2 bell peppers, halved and seeds removed
- 1/2 cup cooked quinoa
- 1/4 cup black beans, drained and rinsed

- 1/4 cup corn kernels
- 1/4 cup diced tomatoes
- 1/4 teaspoon cumin
- 1/4 teaspoon paprika
- Salt and pepper to taste
- 2 tablespoons chopped cilantro
- 2 tablespoons lime juice

Instructions:
1. Preheat oven to 350°F (175°C).
2. In a bowl, mix quinoa, black beans, corn, tomatoes, cumin, paprika, salt, pepper, cilantro, and lime juice.
3. Stuff the bell pepper halves with the quinoa mixture.
4. Place stuffed peppers on a baking sheet and bake for 25-30 minutes, or until peppers are tender.

---

3. SALMON AND AVOCADO WRAPS

Ingredients:
- 1/2 avocado, mashed
- 1 teaspoon lemon juice
- 2 whole grain wraps
- 4 ounces smoked salmon
- 1/2 cucumber, sliced
- 1/4 red onion, thinly sliced
- Handful of arugula

Instructions:
1. In a bowl, mix mashed avocado with lemon juice.
2. Spread avocado mixture evenly on each wrap.
3. Top with smoked salmon, cucumber slices, red onion slices, and arugula.
4. Roll up the wraps tightly and cut in half.

4. TURMERIC LENTIL SOUP

Ingredients:
- 1 tablespoon olive oil
- 1 onion, chopped
- 2 carrots, diced
- 2 celery stalks, diced
- 2 cloves garlic, minced
- 1 teaspoon turmeric
- 1/2 teaspoon cumin
- 1/2 teaspoon paprika
- 1 cup red lentils, rinsed
- 4 cups vegetable broth
- 1 can (14 ounces) diced tomatoes
- Salt and pepper to taste
- Fresh cilantro for garnish

Instructions:
1. In a large pot, heat olive oil over medium heat.
2. Add onion, carrots, and celery. Cook until softened, about 5 minutes.
3. Add garlic, turmeric, cumin, and paprika. Cook for another minute.
4. Add lentils, vegetable broth, and diced tomatoes with their juices. Bring to a simmer.
5. Simmer for 20-25 minutes, or until lentils are tender.
6. Season with salt and pepper.
7. Serve hot, garnished with fresh cilantro.

---

5. MEDITERRANEAN CHICKPEA SALAD

Ingredients:
- 1 can (15 ounces) chickpeas, drained and rinsed
- 1 cucumber, diced
- 1 bell pepper, diced

- 1/4 red onion, thinly sliced
- 1/2 cup cherry tomatoes, halved
- 1/4 cup chopped parsley
- 2 tablespoons olive oil
- 1 tablespoon lemon juice
- 1/2 teaspoon cumin
- Salt and pepper to taste
- Feta cheese (optional)

Instructions:
1. In a large bowl, combine chickpeas, cucumber, bell pepper, red onion, cherry tomatoes, and parsley.
2. In a small bowl, whisk together olive oil, lemon juice, cumin, salt, and pepper.
3. Pour dressing over the chickpea mixture and toss to combine.
4. Crumble feta cheese on top, if desired, before serving.

---

6. TURMERIC CHICKPEA SALAD WRAP

Ingredients:
- 1 can (15 ounces) chickpeas, drained and rinsed
- 1/2 teaspoon turmeric
- 1/2 teaspoon cumin
- 1/4 teaspoon paprika
- Salt and pepper to taste
- 2 whole grain wraps
- 1/2 cup mixed greens
- 1/2 cucumber, sliced
- 1/4 cup shredded carrots
- 1/4 cup hummus

Instructions:
1. In a bowl, combine chickpeas, turmeric, cumin, paprika, salt, and pepper.

2. Mash chickpeas slightly with a fork.
3. Spread hummus evenly on each wrap.
4. Top with mixed greens, sliced cucumber, shredded carrots, and seasoned chickpeas.
5. Roll up the wraps tightly and cut in half.

---

7. SWEET POTATO AND BLACK BEAN QUESADILLA

Ingredients:
- 1 large sweet potato, peeled and diced
- 1 tablespoon olive oil
- 1/2 teaspoon cumin
- 1/2 teaspoon paprika
- Salt and pepper to taste
- 4 whole grain tortillas
- 1 can (15 ounces) black beans, drained and rinsed
- 1/2 cup shredded cheese (optional)
- Salsa and avocado for serving

Instructions:
1. Preheat oven to 400°F (200°C).
2. Toss diced sweet potato with olive oil, cumin, paprika, salt, and pepper.
3. Spread sweet potato on a baking sheet and roast for 20-25 minutes, or until tender.
4. Mash half of the black beans in a bowl.
5. Lay out two tortillas and spread mashed black beans evenly on each.
6. Top with roasted sweet potato, whole black beans, and shredded cheese.
7. Place another tortilla on top of each and press down gently.
8. Heat a large skillet over medium heat and cook quesadillas for 2-3 minutes per side, or until golden brown and crispy.
9. Cut into wedges and serve with salsa and sliced avocado.

---

8. LEMON GARLIC SHRIMP WITH QUINOA

Ingredients:
- 1 cup quinoa
- 1 pound shrimp, peeled and deveined
- 2 tablespoons olive oil
- 3 cloves garlic, minced
- 1/2 teaspoon red pepper flakes
- Juice of 1 lemon
- Salt and pepper to taste
- Fresh parsley for garnish

Instructions:
1. Cook quinoa according to package instructions.
2. In a large skillet, heat olive oil over medium heat.
3. Add garlic and red pepper flakes, and cook for 1 minute.
4. Add shrimp to the skillet and cook for 2-3 minutes per side, or until pink and opaque.
5. Stir in lemon juice and season with salt and pepper.
6. Serve shrimp over quinoa, garnished with fresh parsley.

---

9. LENTIL AND VEGETABLE SOUP

Ingredients:
- 1 tablespoon olive oil
- 1 onion, chopped
- 2 carrots, diced
- 2 celery stalks, diced
- 3 cloves garlic, minced
- 1 teaspoon turmeric
- 1/2 teaspoon cumin
- 1/2 teaspoon paprika
- 1 cup dried green lentils, rinsed

- 4 cups vegetable broth
- 1 can (14 ounces) diced tomatoes
- Salt and pepper to taste
- Fresh parsley for garnish

Instructions:
1. In a large pot, heat olive oil over medium heat.
2. Add onion, carrots, and celery. Cook until softened, about 5 minutes.
3. Add garlic, turmeric, cumin, and paprika. Cook for another minute.
4. Add lentils, vegetable broth, and diced tomatoes with their juices. Bring to a simmer.
5. Simmer for 20-25 minutes, or until lentils are tender.
6. Season with salt and pepper.
7. Serve hot, garnished with fresh parsley.

---

10. MEDITERRANEAN QUINOA SALAD

Ingredients:
- 1 cup cooked quinoa
- 1/2 cucumber, diced
- 1/2 bell pepper, diced
- 1/4 red onion, thinly sliced
- 1/2 cup cherry tomatoes, halved
- 1/4 cup Kalamata olives, sliced
- 1/4 cup crumbled feta cheese (optional)
- 2 tablespoons olive oil
- 1 tablespoon lemon juice
- 1/2 teaspoon dried oregano
- Salt and pepper to taste
- Fresh parsley for garnish

Instructions:
1. In a large bowl, combine quinoa, cucumber, bell pepper, red onion, cherry tomatoes, Kalamata olives, and feta cheese.
2. In a small bowl, whisk together olive oil, lemon juice, oregano, salt, and pepper.
3. Pour dressing over the quinoa mixture and toss to combine.
4. Garnish with fresh parsley before serving.

---

11. TURKEY AND VEGETABLE STIR-FRY

Ingredients:
- 1 tablespoon olive oil
- 1 pound turkey breast, thinly sliced
- 1 bell pepper, thinly sliced
- 1 zucchini, thinly sliced
- 1 carrot, thinly sliced
- 2 cloves garlic, minced
- 1 tablespoon soy sauce
- 1 teaspoon honey
- 1/2 teaspoon ginger, grated
- Cooked brown rice for serving

Instructions:
1. In a large skillet, heat olive oil over medium-high heat.
2. Add turkey breast and cook until browned and cooked through, about 5-7 minutes.
3. Add bell pepper, zucchini, carrot, and garlic to the skillet. Cook for another 5 minutes, or until vegetables are tender-crisp.
4. In a small bowl, whisk together soy sauce, honey, and ginger.
5. Pour sauce over the turkey and vegetables, and toss to combine.
6. Serve over cooked brown rice.

---

12. BLACK BEAN AND QUINOA BURGER

Ingredients:
- 1 can (15 ounces) black beans, drained and rinsed
- 1/2 cup cooked quinoa
- 1/4 cup diced red onion
- 1/4 cup diced bell pepper
- 1/2 teaspoon cumin
- 1/2 teaspoon paprika
- Salt and pepper to taste
- Whole grain burger buns
- Lettuce, tomato, avocado, and other toppings of your choice

Instructions:
1. In a large bowl, mash black beans with a fork.
2. Stir in quinoa, red onion, bell pepper, cumin, paprika, salt, and pepper.
3. Form mixture into patties.
4. Heat a skillet over medium heat and cook patties for 4-5 minutes per side, or until browned and heated through.
5. Serve on whole grain burger buns with lettuce, tomato, avocado, and other toppings of your choice.

---

13. SPINACH AND STRAWBERRY SALAD

Ingredients:
- 2 cups baby spinach
- 1/2 cup sliced strawberries
- 1/4 cup sliced almonds
- 2 tablespoons crumbled feta cheese (optional)
- Balsamic vinaigrette dressing

Instructions:
1. In a large bowl, combine baby spinach, sliced strawberries, sliced almonds, and crumbled feta cheese.
2. Drizzle with balsamic vinaigrette dressing and toss to combine.
3. Serve immediately.

---

14. THAI PEANUT CHICKEN BOWL

Ingredients:
- 1 tablespoon olive oil
- 1 pound chicken breast, thinly sliced
- 1 bell pepper, thinly sliced
- 1/2 cup shredded carrots
- 1/4 cup chopped peanuts
- Cooked brown rice
- Fresh cilantro for garnish

Instructions:
1. In a large skillet, heat olive oil over medium-high heat.
2. Add chicken breast and cook until browned and cooked through, about 5-7 minutes.
3. Add bell pepper and shredded carrots to the skillet. Cook for another 5 minutes, or until vegetables are tender-crisp.
4. In a small bowl, whisk together the Thai peanut sauce ingredients.
5. Pour sauce over the chicken and vegetables, and toss to combine.
6. Serve over cooked brown rice, garnished with chopped peanuts and fresh cilantro.

—

15. GREEK YOGURT CHICKEN SALAD

Ingredients:
- 1 cup cooked chicken, shredded
- 1/2 cup Greek yogurt
- 1/4 cup diced celery
- 1/4 cup diced red onion
- 1/4 cup grapes, halved
- 1/4 cup chopped walnuts
- Salt and pepper to taste
- Whole grain bread or lettuce leaves for serving

Instructions:
1. In a bowl, combine shredded chicken, Greek yogurt, celery, red onion, grapes, and walnuts.
2. Season with salt and pepper.
3. Serve chicken salad on whole grain bread or lettuce leaves.

---

16. CHICKEN AND VEGETABLE STIR-FRY

Ingredients:
- 1 lb (450g) chicken breast, thinly sliced
- 2 tablespoons soy sauce
- 1 tablespoon oyster sauce
- 1 teaspoon sesame oil
- 1 tablespoon vegetable oil
- 2 garlic cloves, minced
- 1 onion, sliced
- 1 red bell pepper, sliced
- 1 green bell pepper, sliced
- 1 cup broccoli florets
- 1 cup snap peas
- Salt and pepper, to taste

- Cooked rice, for serving

Instructions:
1. In a bowl, combine sliced chicken breast with soy sauce, oyster sauce, and sesame oil. Marinate for 15-20 minutes.
2. Heat vegetable oil in a large pan over medium-high heat. Add minced garlic and sliced onion, and cook until onion is translucent.
3. Add marinated chicken to the pan and cook until browned and cooked through.
4. Add sliced bell peppers, broccoli florets, and snap peas to the pan. Cook for another 5-7 minutes, or until vegetables are tender-crisp.
5. Season with salt and pepper to taste.
6. Serve the stir-fry over cooked rice.

17. SALMON SALAD WITH AVOCADO DRESSING

Ingredients:
- 1 lb (450g) salmon fillets
- 2 tablespoons olive oil
- Salt and pepper, to taste
- 6 cups mixed salad greens
- 1 cucumber, sliced
- 1 cup cherry tomatoes, halved
- 1/4 cup red onion, thinly sliced
- 1 avocado, diced

For the Avocado Dressing:
- 1 ripe avocado
- 1/4 cup plain Greek yogurt
- 2 tablespoons lemon juice
- 1 garlic clove, minced
- 2 tablespoons olive oil
- Salt and pepper, to taste

Instructions:

1. Preheat the oven to 400°F (200°C). Place the salmon fillets on a baking sheet lined with parchment paper. Drizzle with olive oil and season with salt and pepper. Bake for 12-15 minutes, or until salmon is cooked through and flakes easily with a fork.
2. In a large bowl, combine mixed salad greens, sliced cucumber, halved cherry tomatoes, thinly sliced red onion, and diced avocado.
3. In a blender or food processor, combine the flesh of one avocado, Greek yogurt, lemon juice, minced garlic, olive oil, salt, and pepper. Blend until smooth and creamy.
4. Serve the salmon over the salad greens and drizzle with the avocado dressing.---

18. TURKEY AND BLACK BEAN WRAP

Ingredients:
- 1 lb (450g) ground turkey
- 1 tablespoon olive oil
- 1 onion, chopped
- 2 garlic cloves, minced
- 1 teaspoon ground cumin
- 1 teaspoon chili powder
- 1/2 teaspoon paprika
- Salt and pepper, to taste
- 1 can (15 oz) black beans, drained and rinsed
- 1/2 cup salsa
- 4 large whole wheat tortillas
- 1 cup shredded lettuce
- 1/2 cup shredded cheddar cheese
- 1/4 cup chopped fresh cilantro
- Greek yogurt or sour cream, for serving (optional)

Instructions:
1. Heat olive oil in a large skillet over medium heat. Add chopped onion and minced garlic, and cook until onion is soft and translucent.

2. Add ground turkey to the skillet and cook until browned, breaking it up with a spoon.
3. Stir in ground cumin, chili powder, paprika, salt, and pepper.
4. Add black beans and salsa to the skillet. Cook for another 5 minutes, or until heated through.
5. To assemble the wraps, place a large whole wheat tortilla on a flat surface. Spoon some of the turkey and black bean mixture onto the tortilla.
6. Top with shredded lettuce, shredded cheddar cheese, and chopped fresh cilantro.
7. Roll up the tortilla, tucking in the sides as you go.
8. Serve the wraps with Greek yogurt or sour cream, if desired.

---

19. SPINACH AND MUSHROOM QUICHE

Ingredients:
- 1 refrigerated pie crust (9 inches)
- 1 tablespoon olive oil
- 1 onion, chopped
- 8 oz (225g) mushrooms, sliced
- 2 cups fresh spinach
- 4 large eggs
- 1 cup milk
- 1/2 cup shredded cheddar cheese
- Salt and pepper, to taste
- Pinch of nutmeg (optional)

Instructions:
1. Preheat the oven to 375°F (190°C). Place the pie crust in a 9-inch pie dish and crimp the edges.
2. In a large skillet, heat olive oil over medium heat. Add chopped onion and sliced mushrooms, and cook until softened, about 5 minutes.
3. Add fresh spinach to the skillet and cook until wilted, about 2 minutes. Remove from heat and let cool slightly.

4. In a large bowl, whisk together eggs, milk, shredded cheddar cheese, salt, pepper, and nutmeg (if using).
5. Stir in the cooked vegetables.
6. Pour the egg mixture into the prepared pie crust.
7. Bake the quiche in the preheated oven for 35-40 minutes, or until the filling is set and the crust is golden brown.
8. Let the quiche cool for a few minutes before slicing and serving.

---

20. TURMERIC CHICKEN AND BROCCOLI BOWL

Ingredients:
- 1 lb (450g) chicken breast, cut into strips
- 2 tablespoons olive oil
- 1 teaspoon ground turmeric
- 1 teaspoon paprika
- 1/2 teaspoon garlic powder
- Salt and pepper, to taste
- 4 cups cooked brown rice
- 2 cups broccoli florets
- 1 red bell pepper, sliced
- 1/4 cup soy sauce
- 2 tablespoons honey
- 2 tablespoons rice vinegar
- Sesame seeds, for garnish
- Chopped green onions, for garnish

Instructions:
1. In a bowl, combine chicken strips with olive oil, ground turmeric, paprika, garlic powder, salt, and pepper. Marinate for 15-20 minutes.
2. Heat a large skillet over medium-high heat. Add the marinated chicken strips and cook until browned and cooked through, about 5-7 minutes per side.
3. In the same skillet, add broccoli florets and sliced red bell pepper. Cook for another 5 minutes, or until vegetables are tender-crisp.

4. In a small bowl, whisk together soy sauce, honey, and rice vinegar. Pour over the chicken and vegetables in the skillet.

5. Cook for an additional 2-3 minutes, stirring to coat the chicken and vegetables in the sauce.

6. To assemble the bowls, divide cooked brown rice among serving bowls. Top with the turmeric chicken and vegetable mixture.

7. Garnish with sesame seeds and chopped green onions. Serve hot.

Chapter 5: Anti-Inflammatory Dinner Recipes

1. SWEET POTATO AND BLACK BEAN CHILI

Ingredients:
- 1 tablespoon olive oil
- 1 onion, chopped
- 2 garlic cloves, minced
- 2 sweet potatoes, peeled and diced
- 1 red bell pepper, chopped
- 1 can (15 oz) black beans, drained and rinsed
- 1 can (14 oz) diced tomatoes
- 2 cups vegetable broth
- 1 tablespoon chili powder
- 1 teaspoon cumin
- Salt and pepper, to taste
- Avocado, cilantro, and lime wedges for serving (optional)

Instructions:
1. In a large pot, heat olive oil over medium heat. Add onion and garlic, and cook until softened.
2. Add diced sweet potatoes and red bell pepper to the pot, and cook for another 5 minutes.
3. Stir in black beans, diced tomatoes, vegetable broth, chili powder, cumin, salt, and pepper.
4. Bring the chili to a simmer and cook for 20-25 minutes, or until the sweet potatoes are tender.
5. Serve the chili hot, topped with sliced avocado, fresh cilantro, and a squeeze of lime juice if desired.

---

2. TURMERIC CHICKEN AND VEGETABLE SOUP

Ingredients:

- 1 tablespoon olive oil
- 1 onion, chopped
- 2 garlic cloves, minced
- 2 carrots, peeled and sliced
- 2 celery stalks, sliced
- 1 teaspoon ground turmeric
- 1/2 teaspoon ground cumin
- 1/2 teaspoon ground coriander
- 6 cups chicken or vegetable broth
- 2 cups shredded cooked chicken breast
- 1 can (15 oz) chickpeas, drained and rinsed
- Salt and pepper, to taste
- Fresh parsley, for garnish

Instructions:
1. In a large pot, heat olive oil over medium heat. Add onion, garlic, carrots, and celery, and cook until softened.
2. Stir in ground turmeric, cumin, and coriander, and cook for another minute.
3. Add chicken or vegetable broth to the pot, and bring to a simmer.
4. Stir in shredded chicken breast and chickpeas, and cook for another 10 minutes.
5. Season the soup with salt and pepper to taste.
6. Serve the soup hot, garnished with fresh parsley.

---

3. LEMON GARLIC SHRIMP WITH ZUCCHINI NOODLES

Ingredients:
- 1 lb (450g) shrimp, peeled and deveined
- 2 tablespoons olive oil
- 4 garlic cloves, minced
- Zest and juice of 1 lemon
- 4 medium zucchinis, spiralized into noodles

- Salt and pepper, to taste
- Fresh parsley, for garnish

Instructions:
1. In a large skillet, heat olive oil over medium heat. Add minced garlic and cook until fragrant.
2. Add shrimp to the skillet and cook for 2-3 minutes per side, or until pink and cooked through.
3. Stir in lemon zest and juice, and season with salt and pepper.
4. Add zucchini noodles to the skillet and toss to combine with the shrimp and sauce.
5. Cook for another 2-3 minutes, or until zucchini noodles are tender.
6. Serve the lemon garlic shrimp over zucchini noodles, garnished with fresh parsley.

4. CHICKEN AND VEGETABLE STIR-FRY

Ingredients:
- 1 lb (450g) chicken breast, thinly sliced
- 2 tablespoons soy sauce
- 1 tablespoon oyster sauce
- 1 teaspoon sesame oil
- 1 tablespoon vegetable oil
- 2 garlic cloves, minced
- 1 onion, sliced
- 1 red bell pepper, sliced
- 1 green bell pepper, sliced
- 1 cup broccoli florets
- 1 cup snap peas
- Salt and pepper, to taste
- Cooked rice, for serving

Instructions:
1. In a bowl, combine sliced chicken breast with soy sauce, oyster sauce, and sesame oil. Marinate for 15-20 minutes.
2. Heat vegetable oil in a large pan over medium-high heat. Add minced garlic and sliced onion, and cook until onion is translucent.
3. Add marinated chicken to the pan and cook until browned and cooked through.
4. Add sliced bell peppers, broccoli florets, and snap peas to the pan. Cook for another 5-7 minutes, or until vegetables are tender-crisp.
5. Season with salt and pepper to taste.
6. Serve the stir-fry over cooked rice.

---

5. TURMERIC SALMON WITH QUINOA AND ROASTED VEGETABLES

Ingredients:
- 4 salmon fillets
- 2 tablespoons olive oil
- 1 teaspoon ground turmeric
- 1 teaspoon ground cumin
- 1 teaspoon paprika
- Salt and pepper, to taste
- 1 cup quinoa, rinsed
- 2 cups water or vegetable broth
- 2 cups mixed vegetables (such as bell peppers, zucchini, and carrots), chopped
- Fresh parsley, for garnish

Instructions:
1. Preheat the oven to 400°F (200°C). Line a baking sheet with parchment paper.
2. Place salmon fillets on the prepared baking sheet. Drizzle with olive oil and sprinkle with turmeric, cumin, paprika, salt, and pepper.

3. Roast salmon in the preheated oven for 12-15 minutes, or until fish flakes easily with a fork.
4. In a medium saucepan, combine quinoa and water or vegetable broth. Bring to a boil, then reduce heat and simmer for 15-20 minutes, or until quinoa is cooked and liquid is absorbed.
5. While the salmon and quinoa are cooking, spread chopped vegetables on a separate baking sheet. Drizzle with olive oil, salt, and pepper. Roast in the oven for 15-20 minutes, or until vegetables are tender.
6. Serve the turmeric salmon with cooked quinoa and roasted vegetables. Garnish with fresh parsley.

6. GINGER TURMERIC CHICKEN STIR-FRY

Ingredients:
- 1 lb (450g) chicken breast, thinly sliced
- 2 tablespoons soy sauce
- 1 tablespoon oyster sauce
- 1 teaspoon sesame oil
- 1 tablespoon vegetable oil
- 2 garlic cloves, minced
- 1 tablespoon ginger, minced
- 1 onion, sliced
- 1 red bell pepper, sliced
- 1 green bell pepper, sliced
- 1 cup broccoli florets
- Salt and pepper, to taste
- Cooked rice, for serving

Instructions:
1. In a bowl, combine sliced chicken breast with soy sauce, oyster sauce, and sesame oil. Marinate for 15-20 minutes.
2. Heat vegetable oil in a large pan over medium-high heat. Add minced garlic, minced ginger, and sliced onion, and cook until onion is translucent.
3. Add marinated chicken to the pan and cook until browned and cooked through.

4. Add sliced bell peppers and broccoli florets to the pan. Cook for another 5-7 minutes, or until vegetables are tender-crisp.
5. Season with salt and pepper to taste.
6. Serve the stir-fry over cooked rice.

---

7. TURMERIC LENTIL SOUP

Ingredients:
- 1 tablespoon olive oil
- 1 onion, chopped
- 2 carrots, peeled and diced
- 2 celery stalks, diced
- 2 garlic cloves, minced
- 1 tablespoon ground turmeric
- 1 teaspoon ground cumin
- 1/2 teaspoon ground coriander
- 1 cup dried lentils, rinsed
- 6 cups vegetable broth
- Salt and pepper, to taste
- Fresh parsley, for garnish

Instructions:
1. In a large pot, heat olive oil over medium heat. Add onion, carrots, celery, and garlic, and cook until softened.
2. Stir in ground turmeric, cumin, and coriander, and cook for another minute.
3. Add dried lentils and vegetable broth to the pot. Bring to a boil, then reduce heat and simmer for 25-30 minutes, or until lentils are tender.
4. Season the soup with salt and pepper to taste.
5. Serve the turmeric lentil soup hot, garnished with fresh parsley.

---

8. MISO-GLAZED SALMON WITH BROCCOLI

Ingredients:
- 4 salmon fillets
- 2 tablespoons miso paste
- 1 tablespoon soy sauce
- 1 tablespoon honey
- 1 tablespoon rice vinegar
- 1 teaspoon sesame oil
- 2 cups broccoli florets
- Cooked brown rice, for serving
- Sesame seeds, for garnish

Instructions:
1. Preheat the oven to 400°F (200°C). Line a baking sheet with parchment paper.
2. In a small bowl, whisk together miso paste, soy sauce, honey, rice vinegar, and sesame oil.
3. Place salmon fillets on the prepared baking sheet. Brush the miso glaze over the salmon.
4. Place broccoli florets on the baking sheet around the salmon.
5. Roast in the preheated oven for 12-15 minutes, or until salmon is cooked through and flakes easily with a fork.
6. Serve the miso-glazed salmon with broccoli over cooked brown rice. Garnish with sesame seeds.

---

9. TURKEY TACO LETTUCE WRAPS

Ingredients:
- 1 lb (450g) ground turkey
- 1 tablespoon olive oil
- 1 onion, chopped
- 2 garlic cloves, minced

- 1 tablespoon chili powder
- 1 teaspoon ground cumin
- 1 teaspoon paprika
- 1/2 teaspoon oregano
- Salt and pepper, to taste
- 1 can (15 oz) black beans, drained and rinsed
- 1 cup salsa
- 1 head iceberg lettuce, leaves separated
- Optional toppings: diced avocado, shredded cheese, Greek yogurt or sour cream

Instructions:
1. In a large skillet, heat olive oil over medium heat. Add chopped onion and minced garlic, and cook until onion is translucent.
2. Add ground turkey to the skillet and cook until browned, breaking it up with a spoon.
3. Stir in chili powder, ground cumin, paprika, oregano, salt, and pepper.
4. Add black beans and salsa to the skillet. Cook for another 5 minutes, or until heated through.
5. To assemble the lettuce wraps, spoon some of the turkey mixture onto each lettuce leaf.
6. Top with diced avocado, shredded cheese, and Greek yogurt or sour cream, if desired.
7. Serve the turkey taco lettuce wraps immediately.

---

10. VEGETABLE AND CHICKPEA CURRY

Ingredients:
- 1 tablespoon coconut oil
- 1 onion, chopped
- 2 garlic cloves, minced
- 1 tablespoon curry powder
- 1 teaspoon ground turmeric

- 1 teaspoon ground cumin
- 1 can (15 oz) chickpeas, drained and rinsed
- 1 can (14 oz) diced tomatoes
- 1 can (14 oz) coconut milk
- 2 cups mixed vegetables (such as bell peppers, carrots, and peas)
- Salt and pepper, to taste
- Cooked rice, for serving
- Fresh cilantro, for garnish

Instructions:
1. In a large pot, heat coconut oil over medium heat. Add chopped onion and minced garlic, and cook until onion is softened.
2. Stir in curry powder, ground turmeric, and ground cumin, and cook for another minute.
3. Add chickpeas, diced tomatoes, coconut milk, and mixed vegetables to the pot. Bring to a simmer and cook for 15-20 minutes, or until vegetables are tender.

---

11. LEMON GARLIC CHICKEN WITH ASPARAGUS

Ingredients:
- 4 chicken breasts
- 2 tablespoons olive oil
- 4 garlic cloves, minced
- Zest and juice of 1 lemon
- 1 teaspoon dried thyme
- Salt and pepper, to taste
- 1 lb (450g) asparagus, trimmed
- Lemon slices, for garnish
- Fresh parsley, for garnish

Instructions:

1. Preheat the oven to 400°F (200°C).

2. Place chicken breasts in a baking dish. Drizzle with olive oil, minced garlic, lemon zest, lemon juice, dried thyme, salt, and pepper. Rub the seasonings into the chicken.

3. Arrange asparagus around the chicken breasts in the baking dish. Drizzle with a little olive oil and season with salt and pepper.

4. Bake in the preheated oven for 25-30 minutes, or until the chicken is cooked through and the asparagus is tender.

5. Serve the lemon garlic chicken with asparagus, garnished with lemon slices and fresh parsley.

12. SWEET POTATO AND KALE SALAD WITH TAHINI DRESSING

Ingredients:
- 2 sweet potatoes, peeled and cubed
- 1 tablespoon olive oil
- Salt and pepper, to taste
- 1 bunch kale, stems removed and leaves torn
- 1/4 cup tahini
- 2 tablespoons lemon juice
- 1 garlic clove, minced
- 2 tablespoons water
- 1/4 cup pumpkin seeds, toasted

Instructions:

1. Preheat the oven to 400°F (200°C).

2. Place sweet potato cubes on a baking sheet. Drizzle with olive oil, salt, and pepper. Toss to coat.

3. Roast sweet potatoes in the preheated oven for 20-25 minutes, or until tender and lightly browned.

4. In a large bowl, massage kale leaves with a little olive oil until softened.

5. In a small bowl, whisk together tahini, lemon juice, garlic, and water to make the dressing.

6. Toss roasted sweet potatoes and kale with the tahini dressing.

7. Sprinkle pumpkin seeds over the salad before serving.

---

13. SPICY SHRIMP STIR-FRY

Ingredients:
- 1 lb (450g) shrimp, peeled and deveined
- 2 tablespoons soy sauce
- 1 tablespoon sriracha sauce
- 1 tablespoon honey
- 1 tablespoon sesame oil
- 1 tablespoon vegetable oil
- 2 garlic cloves, minced
- 1 red bell pepper, sliced
- 1 yellow bell pepper, sliced
- 1 cup snap peas
- Cooked rice, for serving
- Sesame seeds, for garnish

Instructions:
1. In a bowl, combine shrimp with soy sauce, sriracha sauce, and honey. Marinate for 15-20 minutes.
2. Heat sesame oil and vegetable oil in a large pan over medium-high heat. Add minced garlic and cook until fragrant.
3. Add marinated shrimp to the pan and cook for 2-3 minutes per side, or until pink and cooked through.
4. Add sliced bell peppers and snap peas to the pan. Cook for another 5 minutes, or until vegetables are tender-crisp.
5. Serve the spicy shrimp stir-fry over cooked rice, garnished with sesame seeds.

---

14. SPINACH AND MUSHROOM STUFFED CHICKEN BREAST

Ingredients:
- 4 chicken breasts
- Salt and pepper, to taste
- 1 tablespoon olive oil
- 2 cups spinach, chopped
- 1 cup mushrooms, chopped
- 2 garlic cloves, minced
- 1/4 cup grated Parmesan cheese

Instructions:
1. Preheat the oven to 375°F (190°C).
2. Season chicken breasts with salt and pepper. Cut a pocket into each chicken breast.
3. In a skillet, heat olive oil over medium heat. Add spinach, mushrooms, and garlic. Cook until vegetables are tender.
4. Stuff each chicken breast with the spinach and mushroom mixture. Place stuffed chicken breasts in a baking dish.
5. Sprinkle grated Parmesan cheese over the stuffed chicken breasts.
6. Bake in the preheated oven for 25-30 minutes, or until chicken is cooked through.

15. QUINOA STUFFED BELL PEPPERS

Ingredients:
- 4 bell peppers
- 1 cup quinoa, rinsed
- 2 cups vegetable broth
- 1 can (15 oz) black beans, drained and rinsed
- 1 cup corn kernels
- 1 cup diced tomatoes
- 1 teaspoon cumin
- 1 teaspoon chili powder
- Salt and pepper, to taste

- 1/2 cup shredded cheese (optional)
- Fresh cilantro, for garnish

Instructions:
1. Preheat the oven to 375°F (190°C).
2. Cut the tops off the bell peppers and remove the seeds and membranes.
3. In a medium saucepan, combine quinoa and vegetable broth. Bring to a boil, then reduce heat and simmer for 15-20 minutes, or until quinoa is cooked and liquid is absorbed.
4. In a large bowl, combine cooked quinoa, black beans, corn, diced tomatoes, cumin, chili powder, salt, and pepper.
5. Stuff the quinoa mixture into the bell peppers.
6. Place the stuffed bell peppers in a baking dish. If desired, sprinkle shredded cheese on top.
7. Cover the baking dish with foil and bake in the preheated oven for 25-30 minutes, or until the peppers are tender.
8. Garnish with fresh cilantro before serving.

---

16. BUTTERNUT SQUASH AND BLACK BEAN ENCHILADAS

Ingredients:
- 1 butternut squash, peeled, seeded, and diced
- 1 can (15 oz) black beans, drained and rinsed
- 1 onion, diced
- 2 garlic cloves, minced
- 1 teaspoon cumin
- 1 teaspoon chili powder
- Salt and pepper, to taste
- 8 small corn tortillas
- 1 can (15 oz) enchilada sauce
- 1/2 cup shredded cheese (optional)
- Fresh cilantro, for garnish

Instructions:
1. Preheat the oven to 375°F (190°C).
2. In a large skillet, heat olive oil over medium heat. Add diced onion and minced garlic, and cook until onion is translucent.
3. Add diced butternut squash to the skillet. Cook for about 10 minutes, or until squash is tender.
4. Stir in black beans, cumin, chili powder, salt, and pepper. Cook for another 2-3 minutes.
5. Warm the corn tortillas in the microwave or on a skillet to make them pliable.
6. Spoon the butternut squash and black bean mixture onto each tortilla. Roll up and place seam side down in a baking dish.
7. Pour enchilada sauce over the rolled tortillas. If desired, sprinkle shredded cheese on top.
8. Cover the baking dish with foil and bake in the preheated oven for 20-25 minutes, or until enchiladas are heated through.
9. Garnish with fresh cilantro before serving.

---

17. TURMERIC CHICKPEA STEW

Ingredients:
- 1 tablespoon olive oil
- 1 onion, chopped
- 2 garlic cloves, minced
- 1 tablespoon grated ginger
- 1 tablespoon ground turmeric
- 1 teaspoon ground cumin
- 1 can (15 oz) chickpeas, drained and rinsed
- 1 can (14 oz) diced tomatoes
- 4 cups vegetable broth
- 2 cups chopped kale
- Salt and pepper, to taste
- Lemon wedges, for serving

Instructions:

1. In a large pot, heat olive oil over medium heat. Add chopped onion, minced garlic, and grated ginger. Cook until onion is softened.
2. Stir in ground turmeric and ground cumin, and cook for another minute.
3. Add chickpeas, diced tomatoes, and vegetable broth to the pot. Bring to a simmer and cook for 15-20 minutes.
4. Stir in chopped kale and cook for another 5 minutes, or until kale is wilted.
5. Season with salt and pepper to taste.
6. Serve the turmeric chickpea stew with lemon wedges for squeezing over the stew before eating.

---

18. MEDITERRANEAN CHICKEN AND VEGETABLE SKILLET

Ingredients:
- 4 chicken breasts
- 2 tablespoons olive oil
- 1 onion, sliced
- 2 garlic cloves, minced
- 1 red bell pepper, sliced
- 1 yellow bell pepper, sliced
- 1 zucchini, sliced
- 1 cup cherry tomatoes, halved
- 1/2 cup Kalamata olives, pitted
- 1 teaspoon dried oregano
- Salt and pepper, to taste
- Fresh parsley, for garnish

Instructions:
1. Season the chicken breasts with salt and pepper.

2. In a large skillet, heat olive oil over medium heat. Add chicken breasts and cook until browned on both sides and cooked through. Remove from skillet and set aside.

3. In the same skillet, add sliced onion and minced garlic. Cook until onion is softened and fragrant.

4. Add sliced bell peppers and zucchini to the skillet. Cook until vegetables are tender.

5. Stir in cherry tomatoes, Kalamata olives, and dried oregano. Cook for another 2-3 minutes.

6. Return the cooked chicken breasts to the skillet and heat through.

7. Garnish with fresh parsley before serving.

---

19. TURMERIC VEGETABLE PAELLA

Ingredients:
- 2 tablespoons olive oil
- 1 onion, diced
- 2 garlic cloves, minced
- 1 red bell pepper, diced
- 1 yellow bell pepper, diced
- 1 cup cherry tomatoes, halved
- 1 cup green beans, trimmed and halved
- 1 cup frozen peas
- 1 1/2 cups Arborio rice
- 1 teaspoon ground turmeric
- 1/2 teaspoon smoked paprika
- 3 1/2 cups vegetable broth
- Salt and pepper, to taste
- Lemon wedges, for serving
- Fresh parsley, for garnish

Instructions:
1. In a large skillet or paella pan, heat olive oil over medium heat. Add diced onion and minced garlic. Cook until onion is softened.
2. Add diced bell peppers to the skillet. Cook until peppers are tender.
3. Stir in cherry tomatoes, green beans, and frozen peas. Cook for another 2-3 minutes.
4. Add Arborio rice, ground turmeric, and smoked paprika to the skillet. Stir to coat the rice and toast for 1-2 minutes.
5. Pour vegetable broth into the skillet and bring to a simmer. Cook, uncovered, for 15-20 minutes, or until rice is tender and liquid is absorbed.
6. Season with salt and pepper to taste.
7. Serve the turmeric vegetable paella hot, garnished with lemon wedges and fresh parsley.

---

20. GINGER LIME CHICKEN WITH COCONUT RICE

Ingredients:
- 4 chicken breasts
- 2 tablespoons olive oil
- 2 garlic cloves, minced
- 1 tablespoon grated ginger
- Zest and juice of 2 limes
- 1 tablespoon honey
- 1 cup coconut milk
- 1 cup jasmine rice
- 1 1/2 cups water
- Salt, to taste
- Fresh cilantro, for garnish

Instructions:
1. Season the chicken breasts with salt and pepper.
2. In a large skillet, heat olive oil over medium heat. Add minced garlic and grated ginger. Cook until fragrant.

3. Add chicken breasts to the skillet and cook until browned on both sides and cooked through.

4. In a small bowl, whisk together lime zest, lime juice, honey, and coconut milk. Pour over the cooked chicken in the skillet and simmer for 2-3 minutes.

5. In a separate saucepan, combine jasmine rice, water, and a pinch of salt. Bring to a boil, then reduce heat and simmer for 15-20 minutes, or until rice is cooked and liquid is absorbed.

6. Serve the ginger lime chicken over coconut rice, and garnish with fresh cilantro.

Chapter 6: Anti-Inflammatory Snacks and Sides

1. ROASTED GARLIC HUMMUS

Ingredients:
- 1 can (15 oz) chickpeas, drained and rinsed
- 1/4 cup tahini
- 1/4 cup lemon juice
- 2 tablespoons olive oil
- 2 garlic cloves, roasted
- 1/2 teaspoon ground cumin
- Salt and pepper, to taste
- Water, as needed

Instructions:
1. Preheat the oven to 400°F (200°C). Wrap the garlic cloves in foil and roast for 20-30 minutes, or until soft.
2. In a food processor, combine chickpeas, tahini, lemon juice, olive oil, roasted garlic, cumin, salt, and pepper. Blend until smooth.
3. If the hummus is too thick, add water, 1 tablespoon at a time, until desired consistency is reached.
4. Serve the roasted garlic hummus with your favorite vegetables or pita chips.

---

2. BAKED SWEET POTATO FRIES

Ingredients:
- 2 large sweet potatoes, cut into fries
- 2 tablespoons olive oil
- 1 teaspoon paprika
- 1/2 teaspoon garlic powder
- Salt and pepper, to taste

Instructions:
1. Preheat the oven to 425°F (220°C) and line a baking sheet with parchment paper.
2. In a large bowl, toss sweet potato fries with olive oil, paprika, garlic powder, salt, and pepper until evenly coated.
3. Spread the fries in a single layer on the prepared baking sheet.
4. Bake for 25-30 minutes, flipping halfway through, until fries are crispy and golden brown.
5. Serve the baked sweet potato fries hot with your favorite dipping sauce.

---

3. AVOCADO CILANTRO LIME DIP

Ingredients:
- 2 ripe avocados
- 1/4 cup chopped fresh cilantro
- 1/4 cup Greek yogurt
- 1 garlic clove, minced
- Juice of 1 lime
- Salt and pepper, to taste

Instructions:
1. In a bowl, mash the avocados with a fork until smooth.
2. Stir in chopped cilantro, Greek yogurt, minced garlic, lime juice, salt, and pepper until well combined.
3. Serve the avocado cilantro lime dip with vegetable sticks or tortilla chips.

---

4. SPICY ROASTED CHICKPEAS

Ingredients:
- 1 can (15 oz) chickpeas, drained and rinsed
- 1 tablespoon olive oil

- 1 teaspoon smoked paprika
- 1/2 teaspoon cayenne pepper
- 1/2 teaspoon garlic powder
- Salt, to taste

Instructions:
1. Preheat the oven to 400°F (200°C) and line a baking sheet with parchment paper.
2. In a bowl, toss chickpeas with olive oil, smoked paprika, cayenne pepper, garlic powder, and salt until evenly coated.
3. Spread the chickpeas in a single layer on the prepared baking sheet.
4. Bake for 25-30 minutes, shaking the pan halfway through, until chickpeas are crispy.
5. Serve the spicy roasted chickpeas as a crunchy snack.

---

5. STUFFED MINI PEPPERS

Ingredients:
- 12 mini bell peppers, halved and seeded
- 4 oz cream cheese, softened
- 1/4 cup shredded cheddar cheese
- 2 green onions, finely chopped
- 1/2 teaspoon garlic powder
- Salt and pepper, to taste
- Chopped fresh parsley, for garnish

Instructions:
1. Preheat the oven to 375°F (190°C) and line a baking sheet with parchment paper.
2. In a bowl, mix cream cheese, cheddar cheese, green onions, garlic powder, salt, and pepper until well combined.
3. Stuff each mini pepper half with the cream cheese mixture.
4. Place the stuffed peppers on the prepared baking sheet.

5. Bake for 12-15 minutes, or until peppers are tender and cheese is melted.
6. Garnish with chopped fresh parsley before serving.

6. BAKED ZUCCHINI CHIPS

Ingredients:
- 2 zucchinis, thinly sliced
- 2 tablespoons olive oil
- 1/4 cup grated Parmesan cheese
- 1/4 teaspoon garlic powder
- 1/4 teaspoon onion powder
- Salt and pepper, to taste

Instructions:
1. Preheat the oven to 425°F (220°C) and line a baking sheet with parchment paper.
2. In a large bowl, toss zucchini slices with olive oil, Parmesan cheese, garlic powder, onion powder, salt, and pepper until evenly coated.
3. Spread the zucchini slices in a single layer on the prepared baking sheet.
4. Bake for 15-20 minutes, flipping halfway through, until chips are crispy and golden brown.
5. Serve the baked zucchini chips as a healthy snack.

---

7. QUINOA TABBOULEH SALAD

Ingredients:
- 1 cup cooked quinoa
- 1 cucumber, diced
- 1 tomato, diced
- 1/4 cup chopped fresh parsley
- 1/4 cup chopped fresh mint
- 1/4 cup diced red onion
- Juice of 1 lemon

- 2 tablespoons olive oil
- Salt and pepper, to taste

Instructions:
1. In a large bowl, combine cooked quinoa, diced cucumber, diced tomato, chopped parsley, chopped mint, and diced red onion.
2. Drizzle lemon juice and olive oil over the salad. Season with salt and pepper to taste.
3. Toss the ingredients until well combined.
4. Chill the quinoa tabbouleh salad in the refrigerator for at least 30 minutes before serving.

---

8. BAKED SWEET POTATO CHIPS

Ingredients:
- 2 sweet potatoes, thinly sliced
- 2 tablespoons olive oil
- 1/2 teaspoon smoked paprika
- 1/2 teaspoon garlic powder
- Salt and pepper, to taste

Instructions:
1. Preheat the oven to 375°F (190°C) and line a baking sheet with parchment paper.
2. In a large bowl, toss sweet potato slices with olive oil, smoked paprika, garlic powder, salt, and pepper until evenly coated.
3. Spread the sweet potato slices in a single layer on the prepared baking sheet.
4. Bake for 15-20 minutes, flipping halfway through, until chips are crispy and golden brown.
5. Serve the baked sweet potato chips as a crunchy snack.

---

9. GREEK YOGURT DIP WITH VEGETABLES

Ingredients:
- 1 cup Greek yogurt
- 1 tablespoon lemon juice
- 1 tablespoon chopped fresh dill
- 1 garlic clove, minced
- Salt and pepper, to taste
- Assorted fresh vegetables, for serving

Instructions:
1. In a bowl, combine Greek yogurt, lemon juice, chopped dill, minced garlic, salt, and pepper.
2. Stir the ingredients until well combined.
3. Serve the Greek yogurt dip with assorted fresh vegetables like carrots, cucumber, and bell peppers.

---

10. ROASTED CAULIFLOWER BITES

Ingredients:
- 1 head cauliflower, cut into florets
- 2 tablespoons olive oil
- 1 teaspoon smoked paprika
- 1/2 teaspoon cumin
- 1/2 teaspoon garlic powder
- Salt and pepper, to taste

Instructions:
1. Preheat the oven to 425°F (220°C) and line a baking sheet with parchment paper.
2. In a large bowl, toss cauliflower florets with olive oil, smoked paprika, cumin, garlic powder, salt, and pepper until evenly coated.

3. Spread the cauliflower florets in a single layer on the prepared baking sheet.
4. Bake for 20-25 minutes, flipping halfway through, until cauliflower is tender and golden brown.
5. Serve the roasted cauliflower bites as a flavorful side dish or snack.

11. CRISPY BAKED KALE CHIPS

Ingredients:
- 1 bunch kale, stems removed and torn into bite-sized pieces
- 1 tablespoon olive oil
- Salt and pepper, to taste

Instructions:
1. Preheat the oven to 275°F (135°C) and line a baking sheet with parchment paper.
2. In a large bowl, toss kale pieces with olive oil, salt, and pepper until evenly coated.
3. Spread the kale pieces in a single layer on the prepared baking sheet.
4. Bake for 20-25 minutes, or until kale is crispy but not burnt, stirring halfway through.
5. Remove from the oven and let cool before serving.

---

12. CUCUMBER TOMATO SALAD

Ingredients:
- 1 cucumber, diced
- 1 tomato, diced
- 1/4 cup chopped red onion
- 2 tablespoons chopped fresh parsley
- 1 tablespoon olive oil
- 1 tablespoon lemon juice
- Salt and pepper, to taste

Instructions:
1. In a bowl, combine diced cucumber, diced tomato, chopped red onion, and chopped parsley.
2. Drizzle olive oil and lemon juice over the salad. Season with salt and pepper to taste.
3. Toss the ingredients until well combined.
4. Chill the cucumber tomato salad in the refrigerator for at least 30 minutes before serving.

---

13. BAKED PARMESAN ZUCCHINI FRIES

Ingredients:
- 2 zucchinis, cut into fries
- 1/2 cup grated Parmesan cheese
- 1/2 cup panko breadcrumbs
- 1 teaspoon garlic powder
- 1/2 teaspoon dried oregano
- Salt and pepper, to taste
- 1 egg, beaten

Instructions:
1. Preheat the oven to 425°F (220°C) and line a baking sheet with parchment paper.
2. In a bowl, combine grated Parmesan cheese, panko breadcrumbs, garlic powder, dried oregano, salt, and pepper.
3. Dip each zucchini fry into the beaten egg, then coat with the Parmesan breadcrumb mixture.
4. Place the coated zucchini fries on the prepared baking sheet.
5. Bake for 20-25 minutes, flipping halfway through, until fries are golden brown and crispy.
6. Serve the baked Parmesan zucchini fries with your favorite dipping sauce.

---

14. ROASTED RED PEPPER HUMMUS

Ingredients:
- 1 can (15 oz) chickpeas, drained and rinsed
- 1/4 cup tahini
- 1/4 cup lemon juice
- 1/4 cup chopped roasted red peppers
- 2 tablespoons olive oil
- 1 garlic clove, minced
- 1/2 teaspoon ground cumin
- Salt and pepper, to taste
- Water, as needed

Instructions:
1. In a food processor, combine chickpeas, tahini, lemon juice, roasted red peppers, olive oil, minced garlic, cumin, salt, and pepper. Blend until smooth.
2. If the hummus is too thick, add water, 1 tablespoon at a time, until desired consistency is reached.
3. Serve the roasted red pepper hummus with pita chips or vegetable sticks.

---

15. SWEET POTATO AND BLACK BEAN QUESADILLAS

Ingredients:
- 2 medium sweet potatoes, peeled and diced
- 1 can (15 oz) black beans, drained and rinsed
- 1 teaspoon ground cumin
- 1/2 teaspoon smoked paprika
- Salt and pepper, to taste
- 4 large whole wheat tortillas

- 1 cup shredded cheddar cheese
- 1/4 cup chopped fresh cilantro
- Guacamole and salsa, for serving

Instructions:
1. Preheat the oven to 400°F (200°C) and line a baking sheet with parchment paper.
2. Place diced sweet potatoes on the prepared baking sheet. Drizzle with olive oil and sprinkle with ground cumin, smoked paprika, salt, and pepper. Toss to coat.
3. Roast sweet potatoes in the preheated oven for 20-25 minutes, or until tender and slightly caramelized.
4. In a bowl, mash half of the roasted sweet potatoes. Add black beans, remaining roasted sweet potatoes, and chopped cilantro. Mix until combined.
5. Heat a large skillet over medium heat. Place one tortilla in the skillet and sprinkle with shredded cheddar cheese. Spoon sweet potato and black bean mixture over the cheese. Top with another tortilla.
6. Cook quesadilla for 2-3 minutes per side, or until cheese is melted and tortillas are golden brown and crispy.
7. Repeat with remaining tortillas and filling.
8. Serve the sweet potato and black bean quesadillas with guacamole, salsa, and additional cilantro.

16. ROASTED RED PEPPER HUMMUS

Ingredients:
- 1 can (15 oz) chickpeas, drained and rinsed
- 1/2 cup roasted red peppers
- 1/4 cup tahini
- 1/4 cup lemon juice
- 2 tablespoons olive oil
- 1 garlic clove, minced
- 1/2 teaspoon cumin
- Salt and pepper, to taste

Instructions:
1. In a food processor, combine chickpeas, roasted red peppers, tahini, lemon juice, olive oil, minced garlic, cumin, salt, and pepper. Blend until smooth.
2. If the hummus is too thick, add water, 1 tablespoon at a time, until desired consistency is reached.
3. Serve the roasted red pepper hummus with pita bread or vegetable sticks.

---

17. BAKED PARMESAN ZUCCHINI CRISPS

Ingredients:
- 2 zucchinis, thinly sliced
- 1/2 cup grated Parmesan cheese
- 1/2 teaspoon garlic powder
- 1/2 teaspoon onion powder
- Salt and pepper, to taste
- Cooking spray

Instructions:
1. Preheat the oven to 425°F (220°C) and line a baking sheet with parchment paper.
2. In a bowl, combine grated Parmesan cheese, garlic powder, onion powder, salt, and pepper.
3. Dip each zucchini slice into the Parmesan mixture, pressing gently to coat.
4. Place the coated zucchini slices on the prepared baking sheet in a single layer.
5. Spray the zucchini slices lightly with cooking spray.
6. Bake for 15-20 minutes, flipping halfway through, until zucchini is crispy and golden brown.
7. Serve the baked Parmesan zucchini crisps as a crunchy snack.

---

18. SPICY ROASTED CAULIFLOWER

Ingredients:
- 1 head cauliflower, cut into florets
- 2 tablespoons olive oil
- 1 teaspoon smoked paprika
- 1/2 teaspoon cayenne pepper
- 1/2 teaspoon garlic powder
- Salt and pepper, to taste

Instructions:
1. Preheat the oven to 425°F (220°C) and line a baking sheet with parchment paper.
2. In a bowl, toss cauliflower florets with olive oil, smoked paprika, cayenne pepper, garlic powder, salt, and pepper until evenly coated.
3. Spread the cauliflower florets in a single layer on the prepared baking sheet.
4. Roast for 25-30 minutes, stirring halfway through, until cauliflower is tender and caramelized.
5. Serve the spicy roasted cauliflower as a flavorful side dish or snack.

---

19. CUCUMBER AVOCADO ROLLS

Ingredients:
- 1 large cucumber
- 1 avocado
- 1/2 red bell pepper, thinly sliced
- 1/4 cup alfalfa sprouts
- 1 tablespoon lemon juice
- Salt and pepper, to taste

Instructions:
1. Using a vegetable peeler, slice the cucumber lengthwise into thin strips.
2. In a bowl, mash the avocado with lemon juice, salt, and pepper.
3. Spread the mashed avocado onto each cucumber strip.
4. Top with red bell pepper slices and alfalfa sprouts.
5. Roll up the cucumber strips and secure with toothpicks if needed.
6. Serve the cucumber avocado rolls as a refreshing and healthy snack.

---

20. BAKED APPLE CHIPS

Ingredients:
- 2 apples, thinly sliced
- 1 teaspoon cinnamon
- Cooking spray

Instructions:
1. Preheat the oven to 200°F (95°C) and line a baking sheet with parchment paper.
2. Arrange the apple slices in a single layer on the prepared baking sheet.
3. Sprinkle cinnamon over the apple slices.
4. Bake for 1.5 to 2 hours, flipping halfway through, until the apples are dried and slightly crispy.
5. Let the baked apple chips cool completely before serving.

Chapter 7: Anti-Inflammatory Dessert Recipes

1. CHOCOLATE AVOCADO MOUSSE

Ingredients:
- 2 ripe avocados
- 1/2 cup cocoa powder
- 1/2 cup maple syrup or honey
- 1 teaspoon vanilla extract
- Pinch of salt
- Fresh berries, for garnish

Instructions:
1. Scoop the flesh of the avocados into a blender or food processor.
2. Add cocoa powder, maple syrup or honey, vanilla extract, and a pinch of salt.
3. Blend until smooth and creamy, scraping down the sides as needed.
4. Spoon the mousse into serving dishes and refrigerate for at least 30 minutes.
5. Garnish with fresh berries before serving.

---

2. BANANA OATMEAL COOKIES

Ingredients:
- 2 ripe bananas, mashed
- 1 cup rolled oats
- 1/4 cup raisins or chocolate chips
- 1/4 cup chopped nuts (optional)
- 1/2 teaspoon cinnamon
- Pinch of salt

Instructions:

1. Preheat the oven to 350°F (175°C) and line a baking sheet with parchment paper.
2. In a bowl, combine mashed bananas, rolled oats, raisins or chocolate chips, chopped nuts, cinnamon, and a pinch of salt.
3. Drop spoonfuls of the mixture onto the prepared baking sheet.
4. Flatten each cookie with the back of a spoon.
5. Bake for 15-20 minutes, or until the cookies are golden brown.
6. Let the cookies cool on the baking sheet for 5 minutes before transferring to a wire rack to cool completely.

---

3. COCONUT CHIA PUDDING

Ingredients:
- 1/4 cup chia seeds
- 1 cup coconut milk
- 1 tablespoon maple syrup or honey
- 1/2 teaspoon vanilla extract
- Fresh berries, for topping

Instructions:
1. In a bowl, combine chia seeds, coconut milk, maple syrup or honey, and vanilla extract.
2. Stir well to combine.
3. Cover and refrigerate for at least 2 hours, or overnight, until the mixture thickens and sets.
4. Serve the chia pudding topped with fresh berries.

---

4. MIXED BERRY SORBET

Ingredients:
- 4 cups mixed berries (such as strawberries, blueberries, raspberries)

- 1/4 cup honey or agave syrup
- 1 tablespoon lemon juice

Instructions:
1. Place the mixed berries, honey or agave syrup, and lemon juice in a blender or food processor.
2. Blend until smooth.
3. Pour the mixture into a shallow dish and freeze for about 2 hours, or until partially frozen.
4. Remove from the freezer and scrape the mixture with a fork to break up any ice crystals.
5. Return to the freezer for another 1-2 hours, or until firm.
6. Serve the mixed berry sorbet topped with fresh berries.

---

5. CHIA SEED PUDDING

Ingredients:
- 1/4 cup chia seeds
- 1 cup almond milk (or any milk of choice)
- 1 tablespoon maple syrup or honey
- 1/2 teaspoon vanilla extract
- Fresh fruit, for topping

Instructions:
1. In a bowl, combine chia seeds, almond milk, maple syrup or honey, and vanilla extract.
2. Stir well to combine.
3. Cover and refrigerate for at least 2 hours, or overnight, until the mixture thickens and sets.
4. Serve the chia seed pudding topped with fresh fruit.

---

6. BAKED APPLES

Ingredients:
- 4 apples, cored
- 1/4 cup chopped nuts (such as walnuts or pecans)
- 1/4 cup dried fruit (such as raisins or cranberries)
- 1 tablespoon maple syrup or honey
- 1 teaspoon cinnamon
- Pinch of nutmeg

Instructions:
1. Preheat the oven to 375°F (190°C).
2. In a bowl, combine chopped nuts, dried fruit, maple syrup or honey, cinnamon, and nutmeg.
3. Stuff each cored apple with the nut mixture.
4. Place the stuffed apples in a baking dish and cover with foil.
5. Bake for 25-30 minutes, or until the apples are tender.
6. Serve the baked apples warm, optionally with a scoop of vanilla ice cream.

---

7. COCONUT BERRY PARFAIT

Ingredients:
- 1/2 cup coconut yogurt
- 1/2 cup mixed berries (such as strawberries, blueberries, raspberries)
- 2 tablespoons granola
- 1 tablespoon honey or agave syrup
- Shredded coconut, for garnish

Instructions:
1. In a glass, layer coconut yogurt, mixed berries, and granola.
2. Drizzle honey or agave syrup over the top.
3. Sprinkle with shredded coconut for garnish.

4. Repeat for additional parfaits.
5. Serve the coconut berry parfait chilled.

---

8. PEANUT BUTTER BANANA ICE CREAM

Ingredients:
- 2 ripe bananas, sliced and frozen
- 2 tablespoons peanut butter
- 1 tablespoon cocoa powder (optional)
- Splash of almond milk (or any milk of choice)

Instructions:
1. In a blender or food processor, combine frozen banana slices, peanut butter, cocoa powder, and a splash of almond milk.
2. Blend until smooth and creamy, adding more almond milk if needed.
3. Serve the peanut butter banana ice cream immediately as a guilt-free dessert.

---

9. BERRY CHIA SEED POPSICLES

Ingredients:
- 1/4 cup chia seeds
- 1 cup almond milk (or any milk of choice)
- 2 tablespoons honey or agave syrup
- 1 teaspoon vanilla extract
- 1 cup mixed berries (such as strawberries, blueberries, raspberries)

Instructions:
1. In a bowl, combine chia seeds, almond milk, honey or agave syrup, and vanilla extract. Stir well to combine.

2. Let the mixture sit for about 10 minutes, then stir again to prevent clumping.
3. Add mixed berries to the chia seed mixture and stir to distribute evenly.
4. Pour the mixture into popsicle molds and insert sticks.
5. Freeze for at least 4 hours, or until completely frozen.
6. To remove the popsicles from the molds, run warm water over the outside of the molds for a few seconds.

---

10. APPLE CINNAMON BAKED OATMEAL CUPS

Ingredients:
- 2 cups rolled oats
- 1 teaspoon baking powder
- 1/2 teaspoon salt
- 1 teaspoon cinnamon
- 1/4 cup honey or maple syrup
- 1 1/2 cups almond milk (or any milk of choice)
- 1 egg
- 1 teaspoon vanilla extract
- 2 apples, peeled and diced

Instructions:
1. Preheat the oven to 350°F (175°C) and grease a muffin tin.
2. In a large bowl, combine rolled oats, baking powder, salt, and cinnamon.
3. In a separate bowl, whisk together honey or maple syrup, almond milk, egg, and vanilla extract.
4. Pour the wet ingredients into the dry ingredients and mix until well combined.
5. Fold in the diced apples.
6. Spoon the mixture into the prepared muffin tin, filling each cup to the top.
7. Bake for 25-30 minutes, or until the tops are golden brown and firm to the touch.

8. Let the oatmeal cups cool in the pan for 5 minutes, then transfer to a wire rack to cool completely.

---

11. AVOCADO LIME CHEESECAKE BITES

Ingredients:
- 1 ripe avocado
- 1/2 cup coconut cream
- 1/4 cup lime juice
- Zest of 1 lime
- 1/4 cup honey or maple syrup
- 1 teaspoon vanilla extract
- Pinch of salt
- Crushed graham crackers, for topping (optional)

Instructions:
1. In a blender or food processor, combine ripe avocado, coconut cream, lime juice, lime zest, honey or maple syrup, vanilla extract, and a pinch of salt.
2. Blend until smooth and creamy.
3. Spoon the avocado mixture into mini muffin cups or silicone molds.
4. Sprinkle crushed graham crackers on top, if desired.
5. Freeze for at least 2 hours, or until firm.
6. Remove the cheesecake bites from the molds and let them sit at room temperature for a few minutes before serving.

---

12. CHERRY ALMOND ENERGY BITES

Ingredients:
- 1 cup dried cherries
- 1 cup almonds

- 1/4 cup almond butter
- 1/4 cup honey or maple syrup
- 1/2 teaspoon almond extract
- Pinch of salt
- Shredded coconut, for rolling (optional)

Instructions:
1. In a food processor, combine dried cherries, almonds, almond butter, honey or maple syrup, almond extract, and a pinch of salt.
2. Process until the mixture comes together and forms a sticky dough.
3. Roll the dough into small balls, about 1 tablespoon each.
4. Roll the balls in shredded coconut, if desired.
5. Refrigerate for at least 30 minutes before serving.

---

13. CHOCOLATE PEANUT BUTTER BANANA BITES

Ingredients:
- 2 bananas, peeled and sliced
- 2 tablespoons peanut butter
- 1/4 cup dark chocolate chips

Instructions:
1. Spread peanut butter on half of the banana slices.
2. Top each peanut butter-covered banana slice with another banana slice to create a sandwich.
3. Place the banana sandwiches on a baking sheet lined with parchment paper.
4. Melt the dark chocolate chips in the microwave or on the stovetop.
5. Drizzle the melted chocolate over the banana sandwiches.
6. Freeze for at least 1 hour, or until the chocolate is set.
7. Serve the chocolate peanut butter banana bites chilled.

---

14. MANGO COCONUT CHIA PUDDING

Ingredients:
- 1/4 cup chia seeds
- 1 cup coconut milk
- 1 tablespoon honey or agave syrup
- 1/2 teaspoon vanilla extract
- 1 ripe mango, peeled and diced
- Toasted coconut flakes, for topping

Instructions:
1. In a bowl, combine chia seeds, coconut milk, honey or agave syrup, and vanilla extract.
2. Stir well to combine.
3. Cover and refrigerate for at least 2 hours, or overnight, until the mixture thickens and sets.
4. In a blender or food processor, blend the diced mango until smooth.
5. Layer the chia pudding and mango puree in serving glasses.
6. Top with toasted coconut flakes before serving.

---

15. APPLE NACHOS

Ingredients:
- 2 apples, cored and thinly sliced
- 1/4 cup almond butter
- 1/4 cup granola
- 2 tablespoons chocolate chips
- 2 tablespoons shredded coconut

Instructions:
1. Arrange the apple slices on a serving plate.
2. Drizzle almond butter over the apple slices.

3. Sprinkle granola, chocolate chips, and shredded coconut over the almond butter.
4. Serve the apple nachos immediately.

Conclusion

In conclusion, the "Lupus Recovery Diet Cookbook" is more than just a collection of recipes—it's a guide to transforming your relationship with food and embracing a lifestyle that supports your health and well-being. By incorporating these anti-inflammatory recipes into your diet, you're not only nourishing your body but also taking a proactive step towards managing your lupus symptoms.

Each recipe in this cookbook is thoughtfully crafted to be delicious, satisfying, and packed with ingredients that promote healing and reduce inflammation. From comforting soups to vibrant salads, hearty mains to indulgent desserts, every dish is designed to make you feel good from the inside out.

But beyond the recipes, this cookbook is a testament to the strength and resilience of those living with lupus. It's a reminder that even in the face of adversity, there is always room for joy, creativity, and delicious food. So whether you're newly diagnosed or a long-time warrior, this cookbook is here to support you on your journey to health and vitality.

I hope this cookbook inspires you to get into the kitchen, try new flavors, and nourish your body with love and compassion. May these recipes bring you comfort, joy, and a renewed sense of hope as you embark on your lupus recovery journey.

www.ingramcontent.com/pod-product-compliance
Lightning Source LLC
Chambersburg PA
CBHW081225260726
48653CB00010BB/3811